# 28 DAY ANTI INFLAMMATION DIET

*Delicious Recipes for a Healthier You*

**T. John**

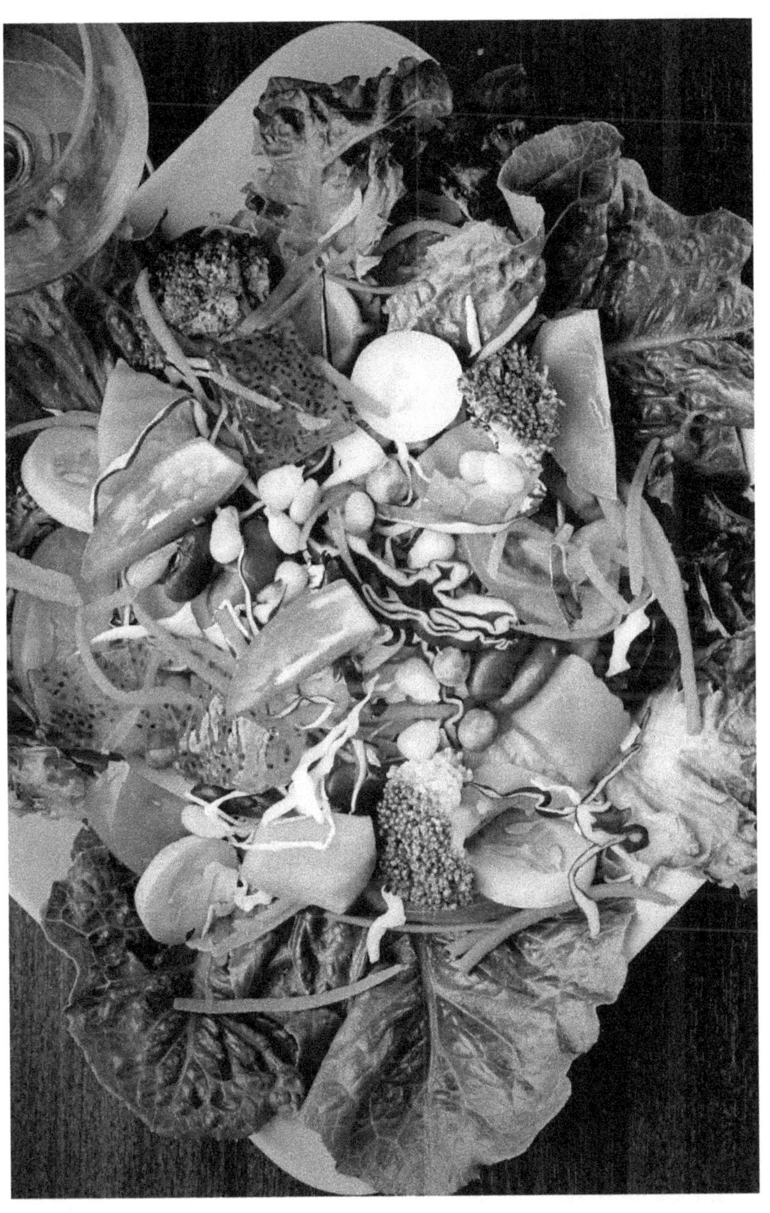

# TABLE OF CONTENTS

## Chapter 5: Snacks and Appetizers ................. 86

# INTRODUCTION

I magine your body as a bustling city. Cells are citizens, proteins are bustling markets, and nutrients are the lifeblood pulsing through its veins. Yet, sometimes, a shadow falls – inflammation, the fiery dragon of the body's defense system.

Inflammation, in its acute form, is a heroic protector. It rallies white blood cells like valiant knights, barricading injured tissues and fending off invaders like viruses or bacteria. But when this fire rages uncontrolled, becoming chronic, the city suffers. It's like dragons torching buildings and roads, leaving behind smoldering ruins of cellular damage.

This chronic inflammation lurks at the heart of many modern maladies, from arthritis and autoimmunity to heart disease and even depression. So, what can we do to tame the dragon, to nurture a city where vibrant health can flourish? Here's where the magic of anti-inflammatory eating kicks in.

It's not about wielding swords or casting spells, but about mindful feasting on nature's bounty. Think of colorful fruits and vegetables, bursting with antioxidants like squelching water buckets on the flames. They're packed with vitamins C and E, carotenoids, and polyphenols – nature's firefighting brigade. Leafy greens, berries, and cruciferous vegetables like kale and broccoli become fortresses against free radicals, the mischievous sparks that ignite the inflammatory inferno.

Fatty fish, like salmon and sardines, add another layer of defense. Their omega-3 fatty acids soothe the fire, calming the knights' overzealous attacks on healthy tissues. Nuts and seeds, sprinkled like golden coins on your plate, deliver vitamin E and fiber, further quenching the flames and promoting cellular repair.

Spice up your feast with turmeric, the golden warrior. Curcumin, its star compound, is a potent anti-inflammatory, a fire-tamer extraordinaire. And don't forget the humble olive oil, nature's liquid gold, dripping with inflammation-fighting oleocanthal.

But remember, this isn't just about what you eat, but what you avoid. Refined sugar and processed foods are like kindling to the inflammatory fire. Ditch the sugary sodas and pastries, and instead, embrace whole grains, legumes, and healthy fats. Think lentils and quinoa, brown rice and sweet potatoes, avocados and almonds. They're the city's sturdy stone walls, built to withstand the dragon's onslaught.

Anti-inflammatory eating isn't just a diet, it's a revolution. It's reimagining your plate as a canvas for health, a masterpiece of colorful vegetables, glistening fish, and nourishing whole grains. It's a dance with the dragon, not a battle, a gentle taming of the fire within. So, take a bite, embrace the symphony of nutrients, and let your body sing the song of vibrant health. Remember, every bite becomes a brick in the city walls, every meal a spark of resilience against the fiery shadow.

This is not just another health trend, but a conscious lifestyle choice, a journey towards a future where the dragons of inflammation are not vanquished, but gently guided back to their rightful role – protectors, not destroyers. So, grab your fork, raise a glass of water (the ultimate hydrator!), and embark on this delicious adventure of anti-inflammatory eating. Let's nourish our bodies, build vibrant cities of health, and dance with the fire, not in fear, but in mindful harmony.

# Chapter 1: 28-Day Meal Plan



## Week1:

Day 1:

- Breakfast: Quinoa Breakfast Bowl
- Lunch: Quinoa and Roasted Vegetable Salad
- Dinner: Turmeric Coconut Chicken Curry
- Snack: Guacamole with Veggie Sticks
- Dessert: Berry and Almond Yogurt Parfait

Day 2:

- Breakfast: Avocado and Kale Omelette
- Lunch: Lentil and Kale Soup
- Dinner: Baked Cod with Garlic and Herbs
- Snack: Hummus and Cucumber Bites
- Dessert: Dark Chocolate Avocado Mousse

Day 3:

- Breakfast: Chia Seed Pudding with Berries
- Lunch: Grilled Chicken Salad with Citrus Dressing
- Dinner: Quinoa-Stuffed Acorn Squash

- Snack: Roasted Red Pepper and Feta Dip

- Dessert: Coconut and Mango Chia Pudding

Day 4:

- Breakfast: Turmeric Golden Milk Smoothie Bowl

- Lunch: Sweet Potato and Chickpea Buddha Bowl

- Dinner: Eggplant and Chickpea Tagine

- Snack: Edamame and Sea Salt

- Dessert: Baked Apple with Cinnamon and Walnuts

Day 5:

- Breakfast: Spinach and Feta Breakfast Wrap

- Lunch: Turkey and Avocado Wrap

- Dinner: Cauliflower and Sweet Potato Curry

- Snack: Greek Yogurt and Berry Parfait

- Dessert: Greek Yogurt and Honey Frozen Popsicles

Day 6:

- Breakfast: Blueberry Almond Overnight Oats

- Lunch: Cauliflower and Broccoli Quinoa Bowl

- Dinner: Lemon Herb Grilled Salmon

- Snack: Almond and Apricot Energy Balls

- Dessert: Turmeric and Ginger Infused Fruit Salad

**Day 7:**

- Breakfast: Sweet Potato and Black Bean Breakfast Hash
- Lunch: Mediterranean Chickpea Salad
- Dinner: Ratatouille with Quinoa
- Snack: Caprese Skewers with Balsamic Glaze
- Dessert: Pumpkin Pie Energy Bites


## Week2:

**Day 8:**

- Breakfast: Greek Yogurt Parfait with Walnuts and Honey
- Lunch: Zucchini Noodles with Pesto and Cherry Tomatoes
- Dinner: Thai-Inspired Shrimp and Vegetable Stir-Fry
- Snack: Kale Chips with Parmesan
- Dessert: Mixed Berry Sorbet

Day 9:

- Breakfast: Salmon and Vegetable Frittata
- Lunch: Spicy Tofu Stir-Fry
- Dinner: Mushroom and Spinach Stuffed Chicken Breast
- Snack: Avocado and Tomato Salsa
- Dessert: Almond Flour Banana Bread

Day 10:

- Breakfast: Green Tea and Berry Smoothie
- Lunch: Shrimp and Quinoa Stuffed Bell Peppers
- Dinner: Sweet Potato and Black Bean Enchiladas
- Snack: Turmeric Roasted Chickpeas
- Dessert: Avocado Chocolate Mousse

Day 11:

- Breakfast: Almond Flour Pancakes with Mixed Berries
- Lunch: Tomato and Basil Chickpea Pasta
- Dinner: Teriyaki Tofu and Broccoli
- Snack: Spinach and Artichoke Stuffed Mushrooms
- Dessert: Pistachio and Cranberry Quinoa Bars

Day 12:

- Breakfast: Mango Turmeric Smoothie
- Lunch: Black Bean and Corn Salad with Avocado
- Dinner: Pistachio-Crusted Baked Cod
- Snack: Quinoa and Black Bean Salad Cups
- Dessert: Lemon Poppy Seed Muffins

Day 13:

- Breakfast: Egg and Spinach Breakfast Muffins
- Lunch: Greek Chicken and Vegetable Skewers
- Dinner: Mediterranean Chickpea and Spinach Stew
- Snack: Smoked Salmon Cucumber Rolls
- Dessert: Cinnamon Roasted Sweet Potatoes

Day 14:

- Breakfast: Buckwheat Banana Pancakes
- Lunch: Spinach and Mushroom Quiche
- Dinner: Spaghetti Squash Primavera
- Snack: Mixed Nuts and Seeds Trail Mix
- Dessert: Blueberry Coconut Ice Cream

# Week 3:

Day 15:

- Breakfast: Mediterranean Veggie Omelette
- Lunch: Quinoa and Roasted Vegetable Salad
- Dinner: Walnut-Crusted Chicken with Roasted Vegetables
- Snack: Guacamole with Veggie Sticks
- Dessert: Pomegranate and Walnut Stuffed Dates

Day 16:

- Breakfast: Quinoa Breakfast Bowl
- Lunch: Lentil and Kale Soup
- Dinner: Turmeric Coconut Chicken Curry
- Snack: Hummus and Cucumber Bites
- Dessert: Dark Chocolate Avocado Mousse

Day 17:

- Breakfast: Avocado and Kale Omelette
- Lunch: Grilled Chicken Salad with Citrus Dressing
- Dinner: Baked Cod with Garlic and Herbs
- Snack: Roasted Red Pepper and Feta Dip
- Dessert: Coconut and Mango Chia Pudding

Day 18:

- Breakfast: Chia Seed Pudding with Berries
- Lunch: Sweet Potato and Chickpea Buddha Bowl
- Dinner: Eggplant and Chickpea Tagine
- Snack: Edamame and Sea Salt
- Dessert: Baked Apple with Cinnamon and Walnuts

Day 19:

- Breakfast: Turmeric Golden Milk Smoothie Bowl
- Lunch: Turkey and Avocado Wrap
- Dinner: Cauliflower and Sweet Potato Curry
- Snack: Greek Yogurt and Berry Parfait
- Dessert: Greek Yogurt and Honey Frozen Popsicles

Day 20:

- Breakfast: Spinach and Feta Breakfast Wrap
- Lunch: Cauliflower and Broccoli Quinoa Bowl
- Dinner: Lemon Herb Grilled Salmon
- Snack: Almond and Apricot Energy Balls
- Dessert: Turmeric and Ginger Infused Fruit Salad

Day 21:

- Breakfast: Blueberry Almond Overnight Oats
- Lunch: Mediterranean Chickpea Salad
- Dinner: Ratatouille with Quinoa
- Snack: Caprese Skewers with Balsamic Glaze
- Dessert: Pumpkin Pie Energy Bites

Day 22:

- Breakfast: Sweet Potato and Black Bean Breakfast Hash
- Lunch: Zucchini Noodles with Pesto and Cherry Tomatoes
- Dinner: Thai-Inspired Shrimp and Vegetable Stir-Fry
- Snack: Kale Chips with Parmesan
- Dessert: Mixed Berry Sorbet

Day 23:

- Breakfast: Greek Yogurt Parfait with Walnuts and Honey
- Lunch: Spicy Tofu Stir-Fry

- Dinner: Mushroom and Spinach Stuffed Chicken Breast
- Snack: Avocado and Tomato Salsa
- Dessert: Almond Flour Banana Bread


Day 24:

- Breakfast: Green Tea and Berry Smoothie
- Lunch: Shrimp and Quinoa Stuffed Bell Peppers
- Dinner: Sweet Potato and Black Bean Enchiladas
- Snack: Turmeric Roasted Chickpeas
- Dessert: Avocado Chocolate Mousse


Day 25:

- Breakfast: Almond Flour Pancakes with Mixed Berries
- Lunch: Tomato and Basil Chickpea Pasta
- Dinner: Pistachio-Crusted Baked Cod
- Snack: Quinoa and Black Bean Salad Cups
- Dessert: Lemon Poppy Seed Muffins


Day 26:

- Breakfast: Mango Turmeric Smoothie

- Lunch: Black Bean and Corn Salad with Avocado
- Dinner: Pistachio-Crusted Baked Cod
- Snack: Quinoa and Black Bean Salad Cups
- Dessert: Lemon Poppy Seed Muffins

Day 27:

- Breakfast: Egg and Spinach Breakfast Muffins
- Lunch: Greek Chicken and Vegetable Skewers
- Dinner: Mediterranean Chickpea and Spinach Stew
- Snack: Smoked Salmon Cucumber Rolls
- Dessert: Cinnamon Roasted Sweet Potatoes

Day 28:

- Breakfast: Buckwheat Banana Pancakes
- Lunch: Spinach and Mushroom Quiche
- Dinner: Spaghetti Squash Primavera
- Snack: Mixed Nuts and Seeds Trail Mix
- Dessert: Blueberry Coconut Ice Cream

# Chapter 2: Breakfast Recipes



Embark on a delightful journey through the mornings with our curated collection of invigorating breakfast recipes designed to kickstart your day with flavor, nutrition, and anti-inflammatory goodness.

## Quinoa Breakfast Bowl

Ingredients:

- 1 cup cooked quinoa
- 1/2 cup fresh berries (strawberries, blueberries, or raspberries)
- 1 tablespoon honey
- 1/4 cup chopped nuts (almonds or walnuts)
- 1/2 teaspoon cinnamon

Instructions:

1. In a bowl, combine cooked quinoa, fresh berries, and chopped nuts.
2. Drizzle honey over the mixture and sprinkle with cinnamon.

3. Gently toss the ingredients until well combined.

4. Enjoy the vibrant flavors of this nutritious quinoa breakfast bowl!

Nutrition Information:

- Calories: 300
- Protein: 8g
- Carbohydrates: 45g
- Fat: 10g
- Fiber: 6g
- Antioxidants: High
- Portion Size: 1 Bowl

## Avocado and Kale Omelette

Ingredients:

- 2 eggs
- 1/2 avocado, sliced
- 1/2 cup kale, chopped
- Salt and pepper to taste
- 1 tablespoon olive oil

Instructions:

1.  In a bowl, whisk the eggs and season with salt and pepper.
2.  Heat olive oil in a pan, add chopped kale, and sauté until wilted.
3.  Pour the whisked eggs over the kale and cook until the edges set.
4.  Place avocado slices on one half of the omelette, fold, and cook until eggs are fully set.
5.  Slide the delicious avocado and kale omelette onto your plate.

Nutrition Information:

- Calories: 280
- Protein: 14g
- Carbohydrates: 8g
- Fat: 20g
- Fiber: 5g
- Antioxidants: Moderate
- Portion Size: 1 Omelette

# Chia Seed Pudding with Berries

Ingredients:

- 3 tablespoons chia seeds
- 1 cup almond milk
- 1/2 cup mixed berries (blueberries, strawberries, and raspberries)
- 1 teaspoon honey
- 1/2 teaspoon vanilla extract

Instructions:

1. Mix chia seeds, almond milk, honey, and vanilla extract in a jar.
2. Refrigerate overnight or for at least 4 hours, allowing the chia seeds to absorb the liquid.
3. Before serving, top the pudding with mixed berries.
4. Delight in the rich texture and natural sweetness of this chia seed pudding.

Nutrition Information:

- Calories: 220
- Protein: 6g
- Carbohydrates: 25g

- Fat: 11g
- Fiber: 12g
- Antioxidants: High
- Portion Size: 1 Bowl

## Turmeric Golden Milk Smoothie Bowl

Ingredients:

- 1 frozen banana
- 1/2 teaspoon turmeric powder
- 1/2 cup coconut milk
- 1/4 cup rolled oats
- 1 tablespoon chia seeds
- 1 tablespoon almond butter

Instructions:

1. Blend frozen banana, turmeric powder, coconut milk, rolled oats, chia seeds, and almond butter until smooth.
2. Pour the smoothie into a bowl and add your favorite toppings.

3. Revel in the nourishing and anti-inflammatory properties of this golden milk smoothie bowl.

Nutrition Information:

- Calories: 320
- Protein: 9g
- Carbohydrates: 40g
- Fat: 15g
- Fiber: 8g
- Antioxidants: High
- Portion Size: 1 Bowl

## Spinach and Feta Breakfast Wrap

Ingredients:

- 1 whole-grain tortilla
- 2 eggs, scrambled
- 1 cup fresh spinach
- 2 tablespoons feta cheese, crumbled
- Salt and pepper to taste
- 1 teaspoon olive oil

Instructions:

1. Sauté fresh spinach in olive oil until wilted.
2. In a separate pan, scramble eggs and season with salt and pepper.
3. Lay the tortilla flat, add the scrambled eggs, sautéed spinach, and crumbled feta.
4. Fold the sides and roll to create a delicious breakfast wrap.

Nutrition Information:

- Calories: 320
- Protein: 18g
- Carbohydrates: 22g
- Fat: 18g
- Fiber: 5g
- Antioxidants: Moderate
- Portion Size: 1 Wrap

## Blueberry Almond Overnight Oats

Ingredients:

- 1/2 cup rolled oats
- 1/2 cup almond milk

- 1/4 cup Greek yogurt
- 1/2 cup fresh blueberries
- 1 tablespoon almond butter
- 1 teaspoon honey

Instructions:

1. Combine rolled oats, almond milk, Greek yogurt, and almond butter in a jar.
2. Stir well and refrigerate overnight.
3. In the morning, top with fresh blueberries and a drizzle of honey.
4. Savor the creamy texture and delightful sweetness of these overnight oats.

Nutrition Information:

- Calories: 280
- Protein: 11g
- Carbohydrates: 32g
- Fat: 12g
- Fiber: 7g
- Antioxidants: High
- Portion Size: 1 Bowl

# Sweet Potato and Black Bean Breakfast Hash

Ingredients:

- 1 sweet potato, diced
- 1/2 cup black beans, cooked
- 1 bell pepper, chopped
- 1/2 onion, diced
- 2 tablespoons olive oil
- 1 teaspoon cumin
- Salt and pepper to taste

Instructions:

1. In a skillet, heat olive oil and sauté diced sweet potatoes until golden.
2. Add chopped onions and bell peppers, cooking until softened.
3. Stir in cooked black beans, cumin, salt, and pepper.
4. Cook until the flavors meld, creating a satisfying sweet potato and black bean hash.

Nutrition Information:

- Calories: 290

- Protein: 9g

- Carbohydrates: 42g

- Fat: 10g

- Fiber: 10g

- Antioxidants: Moderate

- Portion Size: 1 Serving

## Greek Yogurt Parfait with Walnuts and Honey

Ingredients:

- 1 cup Greek yogurt

- 1/4 cup walnuts, chopped

- 1/2 cup mixed berries

- 1 tablespoon honey

Instructions:

1. In a glass, layer Greek yogurt, mixed berries, and chopped walnuts.

2. Drizzle honey over the top for a touch of natural sweetness.

3.  Dive into the layers of this parfait, combining creamy yogurt, crunchy walnuts, and juicy berries.

Nutrition Information:

- Calories: 280
- Protein: 15g
- Carbohydrates: 25g
- Fat: 14g
- Fiber: 5g
- Antioxidants: High
- Portion Size: 1 Parfait

## Salmon and Vegetable Frittata

Ingredients:

- 4 eggs
- 1/2 cup cooked salmon, flaked
- 1 cup mixed vegetables (bell peppers, spinach, tomatoes)
- 1/4 cup feta cheese, crumbled
- Salt and pepper to taste
- 1 tablespoon olive oil

Instructions:

1. Preheat the oven broiler.
2. In an oven-safe skillet, sauté mixed vegetables in olive oil until tender.
3. Whisk eggs, season with salt and pepper, and pour over the vegetables.
4. Add flaked salmon and crumbled feta to the egg mixture.
5. Cook on the stovetop until the edges set, then broil until the top is golden.
6. Slice into wedges and relish the goodness of this salmon and vegetable frittata.

Nutrition Information:

- Calories: 320
- Protein: 22g
- Carbohydrates: 8g
- Fat: 22g
- Fiber: 3g
- Antioxidants: Moderate
- Portion Size: 1 Slice

# Green Tea and Berry Smoothie

Ingredients:

- 1 cup green tea, brewed and cooled
- 1/2 cup mixed berries (strawberries, blueberries, raspberries)
- 1/2 banana, frozen
- 1 tablespoon chia seeds
- 1 tablespoon honey

Instructions:

1. Blend green tea, mixed berries, frozen banana, chia seeds, and honey until smooth.
2. Pour into a glass and enjoy the refreshing taste of this green tea and berry smoothie.

Nutrition Information:

- Calories: 150
- Protein: 3g
- Carbohydrates: 30g
- Fat: 2g
- Fiber: 6g
- Antioxidants: High

- Portion Size: 1 Smoothie

## Almond Flour Pancakes with Mixed Berries

Ingredients:

- 1 cup almond flour
- 2 eggs
- 1/2 cup almond milk
- 1 teaspoon baking powder
- 1/2 teaspoon vanilla extract
- Mixed berries for topping

Instructions:

1. In a bowl, whisk almond flour, eggs, almond milk, baking powder, and vanilla extract until well combined.
2. Heat a skillet over medium heat and spoon batter to form pancakes.
3. Cook until bubbles appear on the surface, then flip and cook the other side.

4. Top with mixed berries and savor the light and fluffy
   texture of these almond flour pancakes.

Nutrition Information:

- Calories: 280
- Protein: 12g
- Carbohydrates: 15g
- Fat: 20g
- Fiber: 5g
- Antioxidants: Moderate
- Portion Size: 3 Pancakes

# Mango Turmeric Smoothie

Ingredients:

- 1 cup frozen mango chunks
- 1/2 teaspoon turmeric powder
- 1/2 cup coconut water
- 1/4 cup Greek yogurt
- 1 tablespoon chia seeds

Instructions:

1. Blend frozen mango chunks, turmeric powder, coconut water, Greek yogurt, and chia seeds until smooth.

2. Pour into a glass and indulge in the tropical goodness of this mango turmeric smoothie.

Nutrition Information:

- Calories: 220
- Protein: 8g
- Carbohydrates: 30g
- Fat: 8g
- Fiber: 6g
- Antioxidants: High
- Portion Size: 1 Smoothie

## Egg and Spinach Breakfast Muffins

Ingredients:

- 4 eggs
- 1 cup fresh spinach, chopped
- 1/4 cup feta cheese, crumbled
- 1/2 cup cherry tomatoes, halved

- Salt and pepper to taste
- Cooking spray

Instructions:

1. Preheat the oven to 350°F (175°C) and grease a muffin tin with cooking spray.
2. In a bowl, whisk eggs and season with salt and pepper.
3. Add chopped spinach, feta cheese, and cherry tomatoes to the eggs. Mix well.
4. Pour the mixture into the muffin tin, filling each cup almost to the top.
5. Bake for 15-20 minutes or until the muffins are set.
6. Allow them to cool slightly before enjoying these flavorful egg and spinach breakfast muffins.

Nutrition Information:
- Calories: 200
- Protein: 15g
- Carbohydrates: 5g
- Fat: 14g
- Fiber: 2g

- Antioxidants: Moderate
- Portion Size: 2 Muffins

## Buckwheat Banana Pancakes

Ingredients:

- 1 cup buckwheat flour
- 1 ripe banana, mashed
- 1 cup almond milk
- 1 teaspoon baking powder
- 1/2 teaspoon cinnamon
- Mixed berries for topping

Instructions:

1. In a bowl, combine buckwheat flour, mashed banana, almond milk, baking powder, and cinnamon.
2. Heat a skillet over medium heat and spoon batter to form pancakes.
3. Cook until the edges are set, then flip and cook the other side.
4. Top with mixed berries and relish the wholesome goodness of these buckwheat banana pancakes.

Nutrition Information:

- Calories: 250
- Protein: 8g
- Carbohydrates: 40g
- Fat: 6g
- Fiber: 6g
- Antioxidants: Moderate
- Portion Size: 3 Pancakes

## Mediterranean Veggie Omelette

Ingredients:

- 3 eggs
- 1/4 cup red bell pepper, diced
- 1/4 cup cherry tomatoes, halved
- 2 tablespoons black olives, sliced
- 1/4 cup feta cheese, crumbled
- Fresh basil for garnish
- Salt and pepper to taste
- 1 tablespoon olive oil

Instructions:

1. In a bowl, whisk eggs and season with salt and pepper.
2. Heat olive oil in a skillet over medium heat.
3. Pour whisked eggs into the skillet, swirling to spread evenly.
4. Sprinkle diced bell pepper, cherry tomatoes, black olives, and crumbled feta on one half of the omelette.
5. Fold the other half over the veggies and cook until the eggs are fully set.
6. Garnish with fresh basil and savor the Mediterranean flavors of this veggie omelette.

Nutrition Information:

- Calories: 280
- Protein: 18g
- Carbohydrates: 6g
- Fat: 20g
- Fiber: 2g
- Antioxidants: Moderate
- Portion Size: 1 Omelette

# Chapter 3: Lunch Recipes

These vibrant dishes are brimming with flavors that will elevate your lunchtime experience. From nourishing salads to hearty bowls and satisfying wraps, each recipe is a symphony of wholesome ingredients designed to contribute to your 28-day anti-inflammatory journey.

## Quinoa and Roasted Vegetable Salad

Ingredients:

- 1 cup quinoa, cooked
- 2 cups mixed roasted vegetables (bell peppers, zucchini, cherry tomatoes)
- 1/4 cup feta cheese, crumbled
- 2 tablespoons olive oil
- Salt and pepper to taste

Instructions:

1. In a large bowl, combine cooked quinoa and roasted vegetables.

2.  Drizzle olive oil over the mixture and toss gently.

3.  Sprinkle crumbled feta cheese on top.

4.  Season with salt and pepper according to your taste.

5.  Serve chilled.

Nutrition Information:

- Calories: 350

- Protein: 10g

- Carbohydrates: 45g

- Fat: 15g

- Fiber: 8g

- Antioxidants: High

- Portion Size: 1 serving

## Lentil and Kale Soup

Ingredients:

- 1 cup dried green lentils, rinsed

- 1 bunch kale, chopped

- 1 onion, diced

- 2 carrots, sliced

- 3 cloves garlic, minced

- 6 cups vegetable broth

- 1 teaspoon cumin
- Salt and pepper to taste

Instructions:

1. In a large pot, combine lentils, kale, onion, carrots, and garlic.
2. Add vegetable broth, cumin, salt, and pepper.
3. Simmer on low heat until lentils are tender.
4. Adjust seasonings to your liking.
5. Serve hot.

Nutrition Information:

- Calories: 280
- Protein: 18g
- Carbohydrates: 50g
- Fat: 2g
- Fiber: 14g
- Antioxidants: Moderate
- Portion Size: 1.5 cups

# Grilled Chicken Salad with Citrus Dressing

Ingredients:

- 2 boneless, skinless chicken breasts
- 4 cups mixed salad greens
- 1 orange, peeled and segmented
- 1/4 cup almonds, sliced
- For the dressing: 2 tablespoons olive oil, 1 tablespoon orange juice, salt, and pepper

Instructions:

1. Grill chicken breasts until fully cooked.
2. Slice grilled chicken into strips.
3. In a large bowl, combine salad greens, orange segments, and sliced almonds.
4. Whisk together olive oil, orange juice, salt, and pepper for the dressing.
5. Drizzle the dressing over the salad and toss.
6. Top the salad with grilled chicken strips.
7. Serve immediately.

Nutrition Information:

- Calories: 400
- Protein: 30g
- Carbohydrates: 20g
- Fat: 22g
- Fiber: 6g
- Antioxidants: High
- Portion Size: 1 serving

## Sweet Potato and Chickpea Buddha Bowl

Ingredients:

- 2 cups sweet potatoes, cubed
- 1 can chickpeas, drained and rinsed
- 1 cup quinoa, cooked
- 1 avocado, sliced
- 2 tablespoons tahini
- Salt and cumin to taste

Instructions:

1. Roast sweet potatoes and chickpeas until golden.

2. In a bowl, assemble quinoa, roasted sweet potatoes, chickpeas, and avocado slices.

3. Drizzle with tahini.

4. Season with salt and cumin to taste.

5. Enjoy warm or at room temperature.

Nutrition Information:

- Calories: 450
- Protein: 15g
- Carbohydrates: 60g
- Fat: 18g
- Fiber: 12g
- Antioxidants: Moderate
- Portion Size: 1 serving

## Turkey and Avocado Wrap

Ingredients:

- 8 oz turkey breast slices
- 1 whole wheat wrap
- 1/2 avocado, sliced
- 1 cup mixed greens
- 1 tablespoon Greek yogurt

- Salt and pepper to taste

Instructions:

1. Lay out the whole wheat wrap.

2. Arrange turkey slices, avocado, and mixed greens.

3. Drizzle with Greek yogurt.

4. Season with salt and pepper.

5. Roll the wrap tightly and cut in half.

6. Serve immediately.

Nutrition Information:

- Calories: 320

- Protein: 25g

- Carbohydrates: 30g

- Fat: 12g

- Fiber: 8g

- Antioxidants: Moderate

- Portion Size: 1 wrap

# Cauliflower and Broccoli Quinoa Bowl

Ingredients:

- 1 cup quinoa, cooked
- 1 cup cauliflower florets, steamed
- 1 cup broccoli florets, steamed
- 1/4 cup pine nuts, toasted
- 2 tablespoons lemon juice
- Salt and pepper to taste

Instructions:

1. In a bowl, combine cooked quinoa, steamed cauliflower, broccoli, and toasted pine nuts.
2. Drizzle with lemon juice.
3. Season with salt and pepper.
4. Toss gently to mix.
5. Serve warm.

Nutrition Information:

- Calories: 380
- Protein: 15g
- Carbohydrates: 45g

- Fat: 16g

- Fiber: 9g

- Antioxidants: High

- Portion Size: 1 serving

## Mediterranean Chickpea Salad

Ingredients:

- 1 can chickpeas, drained and rinsed

- 1 cucumber, diced

- 1 cup cherry tomatoes, halved

- 1/2 cup Kalamata olives, sliced

- 1/4 cup red onion, finely chopped

- Feta cheese, crumbled

- Olive oil, lemon juice, oregano, salt, and pepper for dressing

Instructions:

1. In a large bowl, combine chickpeas, cucumber, cherry tomatoes, olives, and red onion.

2. Drizzle olive oil and lemon juice for dressing.

3. Sprinkle with crumbled feta, oregano, salt, and pepper.

4.  Toss gently to combine.

5.  Serve chilled.

Nutrition Information:

- Calories: 320
- Protein: 12g
- Carbohydrates: 40g
- Fat: 15g
- Fiber: 12g
- Antioxidants: Moderate
- Portion Size: 1 serving

## Zucchini Noodles with Pesto and Cherry Tomatoes

Ingredients:

- 2 large zucchinis, spiralized
- 1 cup cherry tomatoes, halved
- 1/4 cup pine nuts, toasted
- Fresh basil leaves for garnish
- For the pesto: 2 cups fresh basil, 1/2 cup Parmesan, 1/2 cup olive oil, salt, and garlic

Instructions:

1. Spiralize zucchinis into noodles.
2. In a blender, combine basil, Parmesan, olive oil, salt, and garlic for the pesto.
3. Toss zucchini noodles with cherry tomatoes and pesto.
4. Top with toasted pine nuts and fresh basil.
5. Serve cold.

Nutrition Information:

- Calories: 290
- Protein: 8g
- Carbohydrates: 12g
- Fat: 25g
- Fiber: 4g
- Antioxidants: High
- Portion Size: 1 serving

## Spicy Tofu Stir-Fry

Ingredients:

- 1 block firm tofu, cubed
- 2 cups broccoli florets

- 1 bell pepper, sliced

- 1 carrot, julienned

- 3 tablespoons soy sauce

- 1 tablespoon sriracha

- 1 tablespoon sesame oil

- 1 tablespoon ginger, minced

- 2 cloves garlic, minced

Instructions:

1. In a wok or skillet, sauté tofu until golden.
2. Add broccoli, bell pepper, and carrot.
3. Mix soy sauce, sriracha, sesame oil, ginger, and garlic for the sauce.
4. Pour the sauce over the tofu and vegetables.
5. Stir-fry until veggies are tender.
6. Serve over quinoa or brown rice.

Nutrition Information:

- Calories: 320

- Protein: 20g

- Carbohydrates: 25g

- Fat: 16g

- Fiber: 8g

- Antioxidants: Moderate

- Portion Size: 1 serving

## Shrimp and Quinoa Stuffed Bell Peppers

Ingredients:

- 4 bell peppers, halved

- 1 cup quinoa, cooked

- 1 pound shrimp, peeled and deveined

- 1 cup black beans, drained and rinsed

- 1 cup corn kernels

- 1 cup salsa

- 1 teaspoon cumin

- Salt and pepper to taste

Instructions:

1. Preheat the oven to 375°F (190°C).

2. In a bowl, combine quinoa, shrimp, black beans, corn, salsa, cumin, salt, and pepper.

3. Stuff bell peppers with the mixture.

4. Bake for 25-30 minutes until peppers are tender.

5. Serve hot.

Nutrition Information:

- Calories: 380
- Protein: 28g
- Carbohydrates: 45g
- Fat: 10g
- Fiber: 9g
- Antioxidants: High
- Portion Size: 2 halves

## Tomato and Basil Chickpea Pasta

Ingredients:

- 8 oz whole wheat pasta
- 1 can chickpeas, drained and rinsed
- 2 cups cherry tomatoes, halved
- 1/4 cup fresh basil, chopped
- 3 tablespoons olive oil
- 2 cloves garlic, minced
- Salt and pepper to taste
- Parmesan cheese for garnish

Instructions:

1. Cook pasta according to package instructions.
2. In a pan, sauté chickpeas, cherry tomatoes, basil, and garlic in olive oil.
3. Toss cooked pasta with the chickpea mixture.
4. Season with salt and pepper.
5. Garnish with Parmesan cheese.
6. Serve warm.

Nutrition Information:

- Calories: 400
- Protein: 15g
- Carbohydrates: 60g
- Fat: 12g
- Fiber: 10g
- Antioxidants: Moderate
- Portion Size: 1 serving

## Asian-Inspired Salmon Bowl

Ingredients:

- 1 cup brown rice, cooked
- 1 lb salmon fillets

- 2 cups bok choy, chopped
- 1 cup snow peas, trimmed
- 1 carrot, shredded
- For the sauce: 3 tablespoons soy sauce, 1 tablespoon honey, 1 tablespoon rice vinegar, 1 teaspoon sesame oil

Instructions:

1. Grill or bake salmon until cooked.
2. In a pan, sauté bok choy, snow peas, and shredded carrot.
3. Mix soy sauce, honey, rice vinegar, and sesame oil for the sauce.
4. Serve salmon over cooked brown rice and sautéed vegetables.
5. Drizzle with the sauce.
6. Enjoy!

Nutrition Information:

- Calories: 420
- Protein: 30g
- Carbohydrates: 45g

- Fat: 16g
- Fiber: 8g
- Antioxidants: High
- Portion Size: 1 serving

## Black Bean and Corn Salad with Avocado

Ingredients:

- 1 can black beans, drained and rinsed
- 1 cup corn kernels
- 1 red bell pepper, diced
- 1/2 red onion, finely chopped
- 1 avocado, diced
- Cilantro for garnish
- Lime vinaigrette: 2 tablespoons lime juice, 3 tablespoons olive oil, salt, and pepper

Instructions:

1. In a large bowl, combine black beans, corn, bell pepper, red onion, and avocado.

2. In a separate bowl, whisk together lime juice, olive oil, salt, and pepper for the vinaigrette.

3. Drizzle the vinaigrette over the salad.

4. Toss gently to coat.

5. Garnish with fresh cilantro.

6. Serve chilled.

Nutrition Information:

- Calories: 340
- Protein: 12g
- Carbohydrates: 45g
- Fat: 16g
- Fiber: 14g
- Antioxidants: High
- Portion Size: 1 serving

## Greek Chicken and Vegetable Skewers

Ingredients:

- 1 lb chicken breast, cut into cubes
- 1 zucchini, sliced

- 1 red onion, cut into chunks

- 1 bell pepper, cut into pieces

- 1/4 cup feta cheese, crumbled

- For the marinade: 3 tablespoons olive oil, 2 tablespoons lemon juice, 1 teaspoon oregano, salt, and pepper

Instructions:

1. In a bowl, combine chicken, zucchini, red onion, and bell pepper.
2. Whisk together olive oil, lemon juice, oregano, salt, and pepper for the marinade.
3. Marinate the chicken and vegetables for at least 30 minutes.
4. Thread onto skewers and grill until cooked.
5. Sprinkle with crumbled feta.
6. Serve warm.

Nutrition Information:

- Calories: 380

- Protein: 30g

- Carbohydrates: 20g

- Fat: 20g

- Fiber: 5g

- Antioxidants: Moderate

- Portion Size: 1 serving

## Spinach and Mushroom Quiche

Ingredients:

- 1 pre-made whole wheat pie crust

- 2 cups spinach, chopped

- 1 cup mushrooms, sliced

- 1/2 cup feta cheese, crumbled

- 4 eggs

- 1 cup milk (dairy or plant-based)

- Salt and pepper to taste

- Nutmeg for a dash of flavor

Instructions:

1. Preheat the oven to 375°F (190°C).

2. Place the whole wheat pie crust in a pie dish.

3. In a pan, sauté spinach and mushrooms until wilted.

4. Spread the sautéed vegetables over the pie crust.

5. Sprinkle crumbled feta on top.

6. In a bowl, whisk together eggs, milk, salt, and pepper.

7. Pour the egg mixture over the vegetables and feta.

8. Grate a dash of nutmeg over the top.

9. Bake for 40-45 minutes or until the center is set.

10. Allow it to cool before slicing.

Nutrition Information:

- Calories: 320
- Protein: 14g
- Carbohydrates: 20g
- Fat: 20g
- Fiber: 3g
- Antioxidants: Moderate
- Portion Size: 1 slice

# Chapter 4: Dinner Recipes

These dishes are carefully crafted to not only satisfy your palate but also contribute to an anti-inflammatory diet. From aromatic curries to savory stuffed delights, each recipe brings together a harmonious blend of flavors and nourishing ingredients.

## Turmeric Coconut Chicken Curry

Ingredients:

- 1 lb boneless, skinless chicken thighs
- 1 can coconut milk
- 2 tablespoons turmeric powder
- 1 onion, finely chopped
- 3 cloves garlic, minced
- 1 tablespoon ginger, grated
- 1 cup cherry tomatoes, halved
- Salt and pepper to taste
- Fresh cilantro for garnish

Instructions:

1. In a pan, sauté onions, garlic, and ginger until fragrant.
2. Add chicken thighs and cook until browned.
3. Stir in turmeric powder and coconut milk, letting it simmer.
4. Toss in cherry tomatoes and season with salt and pepper.
5. Simmer until the chicken is cooked through.
6. Garnish with fresh cilantro.

Nutrition Information:

- Calories: 350
- Protein: 25g
- Carbohydrates: 10g
- Fat: 25g
- Fiber: 3g
- Antioxidants: High
- Portion Size: 1 serving

# Baked Cod with Garlic and Herbs

Ingredients:

- 4 cod fillets
- 4 cloves garlic, minced
- 2 tablespoons olive oil
- 1 tablespoon fresh parsley, chopped
- 1 teaspoon dried thyme
- Salt and pepper to taste
- Lemon wedges for serving

Instructions:

1. Preheat the oven to 375°F (190°C).
2. Place cod fillets on a baking dish.
3. Mix garlic, olive oil, parsley, thyme, salt, and pepper.
4. Spread the mixture over the cod fillets.
5. Bake for 15-20 minutes until the fish flakes easily.
6. Serve with lemon wedges.

Nutrition Information:

- Calories: 220
- Protein: 30g
- Carbohydrates: 2g

- Fat: 10g

- Fiber: 0g

- Antioxidants: Moderate

- Portion Size: 1 fillet

## Quinoa-Stuffed Acorn Squash

Ingredients:

- 2 acorn squash, halved and seeds removed

- 1 cup quinoa, cooked

- 1 cup black beans, drained and rinsed

- 1 cup corn kernels

- 1 red bell pepper, diced

- 1 teaspoon cumin

- 1 teaspoon paprika

- Salt and pepper to taste

- Fresh cilantro for garnish

Instructions:

1. Preheat the oven to 400°F (200°C).

2. Roast acorn squash halves until tender.

3. In a bowl, mix cooked quinoa, black beans, corn, bell pepper, cumin, paprika, salt, and pepper.

4.  Stuff each squash half with the quinoa mixture.

5.  Bake for an additional 15 minutes.

6.  Garnish with fresh cilantro.

Nutrition Information:

- Calories: 320

- Protein: 12g

- Carbohydrates: 60g

- Fat: 4g

- Fiber: 10g

- Antioxidants: High

- Portion Size: 1 stuffed half

## Eggplant and Chickpea Tagine

Ingredients:

- 1 large eggplant, cubed

- 1 can chickpeas, drained and rinsed

- 1 onion, chopped

- 3 cloves garlic, minced

- 1 can diced tomatoes

- 1 teaspoon ground cumin

- 1 teaspoon ground coriander

- 1 teaspoon smoked paprika
- Salt and pepper to taste
- Fresh parsley for garnish

Instructions:

1. Sauté onions and garlic until softened.
2. Add eggplant, chickpeas, diced tomatoes, cumin, coriander, paprika, salt, and pepper.
3. Simmer until eggplant is tender.
4. Garnish with fresh parsley.

Nutrition Information:

- Calories: 280
- Protein: 10g
- Carbohydrates: 45g
- Fat: 8g
- Fiber: 12g
- Antioxidants: Moderate
- Portion Size: 1 serving

# Cauliflower and Sweet Potato Curry

Ingredients:

- 1 cauliflower, cut into florets
- 2 sweet potatoes, peeled and diced
- 1 can coconut milk
- 2 tablespoons curry powder
- 1 onion, finely chopped
- 3 cloves garlic, minced
- 1 tablespoon ginger, grated
- Salt and pepper to taste
- Fresh cilantro for garnish

Instructions:

1. Sauté onions, garlic, and ginger until fragrant.
2. Add cauliflower, sweet potatoes, and curry powder.
3. Pour in coconut milk and simmer until vegetables are tender.
4. Season with salt and pepper.
5. Garnish with fresh cilantro.

Nutrition Information:

- Calories: 300

- Protein: 8g
- Carbohydrates: 40g
- Fat: 14g
- Fiber: 8g
- Antioxidants: High
- Portion Size: 1 serving

## Lemon Herb Grilled Salmon

Ingredients:

- 4 salmon fillets
- Zest and juice of 1 lemon
- 2 tablespoons fresh dill, chopped
- 2 tablespoons fresh parsley, chopped
- 2 cloves garlic, minced
- Salt and pepper to taste
- Olive oil for grilling

Instructions:

1. In a bowl, mix lemon zest, lemon juice, dill, parsley, garlic, salt, and pepper.
2. Marinate salmon fillets in the mixture for 30 minutes.
3. Preheat the grill and brush with olive oil.

4. Grill salmon for 4-5 minutes per side or until cooked through.
5. Serve with additional lemon wedges.

Nutrition Information:

- Calories: 280
- Protein: 30g
- Carbohydrates: 2g
- Fat: 16g
- Fiber: 0g
- Antioxidants: Moderate
- Portion Size: 1 fillet

## Ratatouille with Quinoa

Ingredients:

- 1 eggplant, diced
- 1 zucchini, sliced
- 1 yellow bell pepper, diced
- 1 red onion, sliced
- 2 cloves garlic, minced
- 1 can diced tomatoes
- 1 teaspoon dried thyme

- 1 teaspoon dried rosemary
- Salt and pepper to taste
- Cooked quinoa for serving

Instructions:

1. Sauté eggplant, zucchini, bell pepper, onion, and garlic until softened.
2. Add diced tomatoes, thyme, rosemary, salt, and pepper.
3. Simmer until vegetables are tender.
4. Serve over cooked quinoa.

Nutrition Information:

- Calories: 250
- Protein: 8g
- Carbohydrates: 45g
- Fat: 4g
- Fiber: 12g
- Antioxidants: High
- Portion Size: 1 serving

# Thai-Inspired Shrimp and Vegetable Stir-Fry

Ingredients:

- 1 lb shrimp, peeled and deveined
- 2 cups broccoli florets
- 1 red bell pepper, sliced
- 1 carrot, julienned
- 2 tablespoons soy sauce
- 1 tablespoon fish sauce
- 1 tablespoon honey
- 1 teaspoon ginger, grated
- 2 cloves garlic, minced
- 2 tablespoons sesame oil
- Fresh cilantro for garnish

Instructions:

1. Stir-fry shrimp, broccoli, bell pepper, and carrot in sesame oil.
2. In a bowl, mix soy sauce, fish sauce, honey, ginger, and garlic.
3. Pour the sauce over the stir-fry and cook until shrimp is pink.

4.  Garnish with fresh cilantro.

Nutrition Information:

- Calories: 280
- Protein: 25g
- Carbohydrates: 18g
- Fat: 12g
- Fiber: 4g
- Antioxidants: Moderate
- Portion Size: 1 serving

# Mushroom and Spinach Stuffed Chicken Breast

Ingredients:

- 4 boneless, skinless chicken breasts
- 2 cups mushrooms, chopped
- 2 cups spinach, chopped
- 3 cloves garlic, minced
- 1 teaspoon dried thyme
- 1 teaspoon dried rosemary
- Salt and pepper to taste

- Olive oil for cooking

Instructions:

1. Preheat the oven to 375°F (190°C).
2. Butterfly chicken breasts and season with salt, pepper, thyme, and rosemary.
3. Sauté mushrooms, spinach, and garlic in olive oil.
4. Stuff each chicken breast with the mushroom and spinach mixture.
5. Bake for 25-30 minutes or until chicken is cooked through.

Nutrition Information:

- Calories: 320
- Protein: 30g
- Carbohydrates: 5g
- Fat: 18g
- Fiber: 2g
- Antioxidants: High
- Portion Size: 1 stuffed breast

# Sweet Potato and Black Bean Enchiladas

Ingredients:

- 2 large sweet potatoes, diced
- 1 can black beans, drained and rinsed
- 1 red onion, finely chopped
- 2 teaspoons ground cumin
- 2 teaspoons chili powder
- 8 whole wheat tortillas
- 2 cups enchilada sauce
- 1 cup shredded cheese (optional)
- Fresh cilantro for garnish

Instructions:

1. Roast sweet potatoes until tender.
2. In a bowl, mix sweet potatoes, black beans, red onion, cumin, and chili powder.
3. Spoon the mixture onto each tortilla and roll them up.
4. Place the enchiladas in a baking dish, cover with enchilada sauce and cheese.
5. Bake until the cheese is melted and bubbly.
6. Garnish with fresh cilantro.

Nutrition Information:

- Calories: 350
- Protein: 15g
- Carbohydrates: 60g
- Fat: 8g
- Fiber: 12g
- Antioxidants: Moderate
- Portion Size: 2 enchiladas

## Teriyaki Tofu and Broccoli

Ingredients:

- 1 lb firm tofu, cubed
- 2 cups broccoli florets
- 1 red bell pepper, sliced
- 1/2 cup teriyaki sauce
- 2 tablespoons soy sauce
- 1 tablespoon rice vinegar
- 1 tablespoon sesame oil
- 2 teaspoons cornstarch
- 1 teaspoon ginger, grated
- 2 cloves garlic, minced
- Sesame seeds for garnish

Instructions:

1. In a wok, stir-fry tofu, broccoli, and bell pepper in sesame oil.
2. In a bowl, mix teriyaki sauce, soy sauce, rice vinegar, cornstarch, ginger, and garlic.
3. Pour the sauce over the tofu and vegetables, stirring until thickened.
4. Garnish with sesame seeds.

Nutrition Information:

- Calories: 280
- Protein: 18g
- Carbohydrates: 25g
- Fat: 12g
- Fiber: 6g
- Antioxidants: High
- Portion Size: 1 serving

## Pistachio-Crusted Baked Cod

Ingredients:

- 4 cod fillets
- 1/2 cup pistachios, finely chopped

- 1/4 cup whole wheat breadcrumbs

- 1 teaspoon dried thyme

- 1 teaspoon lemon zest

- Salt and pepper to taste

- Olive oil for baking

Instructions:

1. Preheat the oven to 400°F (200°C).

2. Mix pistachios, breadcrumbs, thyme, lemon zest, salt, and pepper.

3. Coat each cod fillet with the pistachio mixture.

4. Place the fillets on a baking sheet, drizzle with olive oil.

5. Bake for 15-20 minutes or until the fish flakes easily.

Nutrition Information:

- Calories: 250

- Protein: 25g

- Carbohydrates: 10g

- Fat: 12g

- Fiber: 3g

- Antioxidants: Moderate

- Portion Size: 1 fillet

## Mediterranean Chickpea and Spinach Stew

Ingredients:

- 2 cans chickpeas, drained and rinsed
- 4 cups fresh spinach
- 1 can diced tomatoes
- 1 onion, chopped
- 3 cloves garlic, minced
- 1 teaspoon dried oregano
- 1 teaspoon dried basil
- Salt and pepper to taste
- Feta cheese for garnish

Instructions:

1. Sauté onions and garlic until softened.
2. Add chickpeas, diced tomatoes, oregano, basil, salt, and pepper.
3. Simmer until flavors meld.
4. Stir in fresh spinach until wilted.

5.  Garnish with crumbled feta.



Nutrition Information:

- Calories: 300

- Protein: 15g

- Carbohydrates: 45g

- Fat: 8g

- Fiber: 12g

- Antioxidants: High

- Portion Size: 1 serving

## Spaghetti Squash Primavera

Ingredients:

- 1 spaghetti squash, halved and seeds removed

- 1 cup cherry tomatoes, halved

- 1 zucchini, spiralized

- 1 yellow bell pepper, sliced

- 2 tablespoons olive oil

- 2 cloves garlic, minced

- 1 teaspoon dried Italian herbs

- Salt and pepper to taste

- Fresh basil for garnish

Instructions:

1. Roast spaghetti squash until strands can be easily separated.
2. In a pan, sauté cherry tomatoes, zucchini, bell pepper, and garlic in olive oil.
3. Toss in spaghetti squash strands and season with Italian herbs, salt, and pepper.
4. Cook until vegetables are tender.
5. Garnish with fresh basil.

Nutrition Information:

- Calories: 230
- Protein: 3g
- Carbohydrates: 30g
- Fat: 12g
- Fiber: 7g
- Antioxidants: Moderate
- Portion Size: 1 serving

# Walnut-Crusted Chicken with Roasted Vegetables

Ingredients:

- 4 chicken breasts
- 1 cup walnuts, finely chopped
- 1/4 cup whole wheat breadcrumbs
- 1 teaspoon dried thyme
- 1 teaspoon Dijon mustard
- 2 tablespoons olive oil
- Salt and pepper to taste
- Assorted vegetables for roasting

Instructions:

1. Preheat the oven to 375°F (190°C).
2. Mix chopped walnuts, breadcrumbs, thyme, Dijon mustard, olive oil, salt, and pepper.
3. Coat each chicken breast with the walnut mixture.
4. Place the chicken breasts on a baking sheet with assorted vegetables.
5. Roast for 25-30 minutes or until chicken is cooked through.

Nutrition Information:

- Calories: 320
- Protein: 30g
- Carbohydrates: 10g
- Fat: 18g
- Fiber: 4g
- Antioxidants: High
- Portion Size: 1 serving

# Chapter 5: Snacks and Appetizers

In Chapter 5, we embark on a journey through snack and appetizer recipes that not only satisfy cravings but also align with the principles of an anti-inflammatory lifestyle.

## Guacamole with Veggie Sticks

Ingredients:

- 3 ripe avocados
- 1 small red onion, finely diced
- 2 tomatoes, diced
- 1 clove garlic, minced
- 1 lime, juiced
- Salt and pepper to taste
- Assorted veggie sticks for dipping

Instructions:

1. In a bowl, mash the avocados with a fork.
2. Add the diced red onion, tomatoes, minced garlic, and lime juice.
3. Mix until well combined.

4. Season with salt and pepper to taste.

5. Serve chilled with an assortment of veggie sticks.

Nutrition Information:

- Calories: 120

- Protein: 2g

- Carbohydrates: 8g

- Fat: 10g

- Fiber: 5g

- Antioxidants: High

- Portion Size: 1/4 cup guacamole with veggie sticks

## Hummus and Cucumber Bites

Ingredients:

- 1 cup chickpeas, cooked or canned

- 1/4 cup tahini

- 2 cloves garlic

- 2 tablespoons olive oil

- 1 lemon, juiced

- Salt and cumin to taste

- Cucumber slices for serving

Instructions:

1. In a blender, combine chickpeas, tahini, garlic, olive oil, lemon juice, salt, and cumin.
2. Blend until smooth, adding water if needed for consistency.
3. Spread hummus on cucumber slices.
4. Garnish with a sprinkle of cumin.
5. Serve chilled.

Nutrition Information:

- Calories: 90
- Protein: 3g
- Carbohydrates: 9g
- Fat: 5g
- Fiber: 3g
- Antioxidants: Moderate
- Portion Size: 2 cucumber bites with hummus

## Roasted Red Pepper and Feta Dip

Ingredients:

- 2 large red bell peppers, roasted and peeled
- 1/2 cup feta cheese, crumbled

- 2 tablespoons olive oil

- 1 clove garlic, minced

- 1 teaspoon balsamic vinegar

- Salt and pepper to taste

- Pita triangles for dipping

Instructions:

1. Blend roasted red peppers, feta cheese, olive oil, minced garlic, and balsamic vinegar until smooth.
2. Season with salt and pepper to taste.
3. Transfer to a bowl and refrigerate for at least 30 minutes.
4. Serve chilled with pita triangles.

Nutrition Information:

- Calories: 70

- Protein: 3g

- Carbohydrates: 5g

- Fat: 5g

- Fiber: 1g

- Antioxidants: High

- Portion Size: 2 tablespoons dip with pita triangles

## Edamame and Sea Salt

Ingredients:

- 2 cups edamame, steamed and cooled
- Sea salt to taste

Instructions:

1. In a bowl, toss steamed edamame with sea salt.
2. Serve in a bowl for convenient snacking.

Nutrition Information:

- Calories: 120
- Protein: 11g
- Carbohydrates: 8g
- Fat: 4g
- Fiber: 5g
- Antioxidants: Moderate
- Portion Size: 1 cup edamame

## Greek Yogurt and Berry Parfait

Ingredients:

- 1 cup Greek yogurt

- 1/2 cup mixed berries (strawberries, blueberries, raspberries)
- 2 tablespoons honey
- Granola for layering

Instructions:

1. In a glass, layer Greek yogurt, mixed berries, and granola.
2. Drizzle honey over the top layer.
3. Repeat for additional layers.
4. Serve chilled.

Nutrition Information:

- Calories: 180
- Protein: 15g
- Carbohydrates: 25g
- Fat: 3g
- Fiber: 4g
- Antioxidants: High
- Portion Size: 1 parfait

# Almond and Apricot Energy Balls

Ingredients:

- 1 cup almonds, raw and unsalted
- 1 cup dried apricots, pitted
- 1 tablespoon chia seeds
- 1 tablespoon honey
- Shredded coconut for coating

Instructions:

1. In a food processor, blend almonds, dried apricots, chia seeds, and honey until a sticky mixture forms.
2. Roll the mixture into bite-sized balls.
3. Coat each ball with shredded coconut.
4. Refrigerate for 30 minutes before serving.

Nutrition Information:

- Calories: 70
- Protein: 2g
- Carbohydrates: 8g
- Fat: 4g
- Fiber: 2g
- Antioxidants: Moderate

- Portion Size: 2 energy balls

## Caprese Skewers with Balsamic Glaze

Ingredients:

- Cherry tomatoes
- Fresh mozzarella balls
- Fresh basil leaves
- Balsamic glaze for drizzling

Instructions:

1. Thread a cherry tomato, a mozzarella ball, and a basil leaf onto each skewer.
2. Arrange the skewers on a serving platter.
3. Drizzle with balsamic glaze just before serving.

Nutrition Information:

- Calories: 60
- Protein: 4g
- Carbohydrates: 3g
- Fat: 4g

- Fiber: 1g
- Antioxidants: High
- Portion Size: 3 skewers

## Kale Chips with Parmesan

Ingredients:

- 1 bunch kale, stems removed and leaves torn into bite-sized pieces
- 1 tablespoon olive oil
- 2 tablespoons grated Parmesan cheese
- Salt and pepper to taste

Instructions:

1. Preheat the oven to 350°F (175°C).
2. In a bowl, toss kale with olive oil, Parmesan, salt, and pepper.
3. Spread the kale on a baking sheet in a single layer.
4. Bake for 10-15 minutes or until crispy.

Nutrition Information:

- Calories: 80
- Protein: 4g

- Carbohydrates: 6g

- Fat: 5g

- Fiber: 2g

- Antioxidants: Moderate

- Portion Size: 1 cup kale chips

## Avocado and Tomato Salsa

Ingredients:

- 2 ripe avocados, diced

- 1 cup cherry tomatoes, halved

- 1/4 cup red onion, finely chopped

- 1 jalapeño, seeded and finely diced

- Fresh cilantro, chopped

- Lime juice, to taste

- Salt and pepper to taste

- Whole-grain tortilla chips for serving

Instructions:

1. In a bowl, combine diced avocados, cherry tomatoes, red onion, jalapeño, and cilantro.

2. Drizzle with lime juice and gently toss.

3. Season with salt and pepper to taste.

4. Serve with whole-grain tortilla chips.

Nutrition Information:

- Calories: 100

- Protein: 2g

- Carbohydrates: 8g

- Fat: 7g

- Fiber: 4g

- Antioxidants: High

- Portion Size: 1/2 cup salsa with chips

# Turmeric Roasted Chickpeas

Ingredients:

- 2 cans chickpeas, drained and rinsed

- 2 tablespoons olive oil

- 1 teaspoon turmeric

- 1/2 teaspoon cumin

- 1/2 teaspoon smoked paprika

- Salt to taste

Instructions:

1. Preheat the oven to 400°F (200°C).

2. In a bowl, toss chickpeas with olive oil, turmeric, cumin, smoked paprika, and salt.

3. Spread the chickpeas on a baking sheet.

4. Roast for 25-30 minutes or until golden and crispy.

Nutrition Information:

- Calories: 120

- Protein: 5g

- Carbohydrates: 16g

- Fat: 4g

- Fiber: 4g

- Antioxidants: Moderate

- Portion Size: 1/2 cup roasted chickpeas

## Spinach and Artichoke Stuffed Mushrooms

Ingredients:

- 12 large mushrooms, stems removed

- 1 cup frozen spinach, thawed and drained

- 1/2 cup artichoke hearts, chopped

- 1/4 cup cream cheese

- 1/4 cup grated Parmesan cheese

- 1 clove garlic, minced

- Salt and pepper to taste

Instructions:

1. Preheat the oven to 375°F (190°C).

2. In a bowl, mix together spinach, artichoke hearts, cream cheese, Parmesan, garlic, salt, and pepper.

3. Stuff each mushroom cap with the mixture.

4. Bake for 20 minutes or until mushrooms are tender.

Nutrition Information:

- Calories: 90

- Protein: 6g

- Carbohydrates: 7g

- Fat: 5g

- Fiber: 2g

- Antioxidants: Moderate

- Portion Size: 2 stuffed mushrooms

# Quinoa and Black Bean Salad Cups

Ingredients:

- 1 cup cooked quinoa
- 1 cup black beans, cooked and drained
- 1 cup cherry tomatoes, quartered
- 1/4 cup red onion, finely chopped
- 1/4 cup fresh cilantro, chopped
- Lime vinaigrette (lime juice, olive oil, salt, and pepper)
- Boston lettuce leaves for cups

Instructions:

1. In a bowl, combine cooked quinoa, black beans, cherry tomatoes, red onion, and cilantro.
2. Drizzle with lime vinaigrette and toss to coat.
3. Spoon the mixture into Boston lettuce leaves, creating cups.
4. Serve chilled.

Nutrition Information:

- Calories: 150
- Protein: 7g

- Carbohydrates: 25g

- Fat: 3g

- Fiber: 6g

- Antioxidants: High

- Portion Size: 1 cup salad cups

## Smoked Salmon Cucumber Rolls

Ingredients:

- English cucumber, thinly sliced lengthwise

- Smoked salmon slices

- Cream cheese

- Fresh dill, for garnish

Instructions:

1. Lay cucumber slices flat and spread a thin layer of cream cheese.
2. Place a slice of smoked salmon on top.
3. Roll up each slice and secure with a toothpick.
4. Garnish with fresh dill before serving.

Nutrition Information:

- Calories: 60

- Protein: 4g

- Carbohydrates: 2g

- Fat: 4g

- Fiber: 1g

- Antioxidants: Moderate

- Portion Size: 3 cucumber rolls

## Mixed Nuts and Seeds Trail Mix

Ingredients:

- 1 cup mixed nuts (almonds, walnuts, cashews)

- 1/4 cup pumpkin seeds

- 1/4 cup sunflower seeds

- 1/4 cup dried cranberries

- 1/4 teaspoon cinnamon

Instructions:

1. In a bowl, combine mixed nuts, pumpkin seeds, sunflower seeds, dried cranberries, and cinnamon.

2. Toss until well mixed.

3. Portion into snack-sized bags for easy grab-and-go.

Nutrition Information:

- Calories: 180
- Protein: 5g
- Carbohydrates: 12g
- Fat: 14g
- Fiber: 3g
- Antioxidants: High
- Portion Size: 1/4 cup trail mix

## Sweet Potato Fries with Garlic Aioli

Ingredients:

- 2 large sweet potatoes, cut into fries
- 2 tablespoons olive oil
- 1 teaspoon paprika
- Salt and pepper to taste
- For garlic aioli: Greek yogurt, minced garlic, lemon juice, salt

Instructions:

1. Preheat the oven to 425°F (220°C).
2. Toss sweet potato fries with olive oil, paprika, salt, and pepper.

3. Spread fries on a baking sheet and bake for 25-30 minutes or until crispy.

4. Mix Greek yogurt, minced garlic, lemon juice, and salt for garlic aioli.

5. Serve sweet potato fries with garlic aioli for dipping.

Nutrition Information:

- Calories: 160

- Protein: 3g

- Carbohydrates: 26g

- Fat: 5g

- Fiber: 4g

- Antioxidants: Moderate

- Portion Size: 1 cup sweet potato fries with aioli

# Chapter 6: Desserts

Desserts are often considered a guilty pleasure, but fear not – these recipes are crafted to not only satisfy your sweet tooth but also contribute to your overall well-being.

## Berry and Almond Yogurt Parfait

Ingredients:

- 1 cup Greek yogurt
- 1/2 cup mixed berries (strawberries, blueberries, raspberries)
- 2 tablespoons almonds, sliced
- 1 tablespoon honey

Instructions:

1. In a glass or bowl, layer Greek yogurt at the bottom.
2. Add a layer of mixed berries on top of the yogurt.
3. Sprinkle sliced almonds over the berries.
4. Drizzle honey over the top.
5. Repeat the layers if desired.
6. Enjoy!

Nutrition Information:

- Calories: 250
- Protein: 15g
- Carbohydrates: 25g
- Fat: 12g
- Fiber: 5g
- Antioxidants: High
- Portion Size: 1 serving

## Dark Chocolate Avocado Mousse

Ingredients:

- 2 ripe avocados
- 1/4 cup dark cocoa powder
- 1/4 cup maple syrup
- 1 teaspoon vanilla extract
- Pinch of sea salt

Instructions:

1. In a blender, combine avocados, cocoa powder, maple syrup, vanilla extract, and sea salt.
2. Blend until smooth and creamy.
3. Refrigerate for at least 30 minutes before serving.

4. Serve chilled and indulge guilt-free!

Nutrition Information:

- Calories: 220

- Protein: 3g

- Carbohydrates: 20g

- Fat: 15g

- Fiber: 7g

- Antioxidants: Moderate

- Portion Size: 1 serving

## Coconut and Mango Chia Pudding

Ingredients:

- 1/4 cup chia seeds

- 1 cup coconut milk

- 1/2 cup diced mango

- 1 tablespoon shredded coconut

- 1 teaspoon agave nectar

Instructions:

1. Mix chia seeds and coconut milk in a bowl, let it sit for 10 minutes.

2.  Stir the mixture to avoid clumps.

3.  Refrigerate for at least 4 hours or overnight.

4.  Top with diced mango, shredded coconut, and a drizzle of agave nectar.

5.  Dive into this delightful pudding!

Nutrition Information:

- Calories: 180
- Protein: 5g
- Carbohydrates: 20g
- Fat: 10g
- Fiber: 8g
- Antioxidants: High
- Portion Size: 1 serving

## Baked Apple with Cinnamon and Walnuts

Ingredients:

- 2 apples, cored and halved
- 1 teaspoon cinnamon
- 2 tablespoons chopped walnuts

- 1 tablespoon honey

Instructions:

1. Preheat the oven to 375°F (190°C).
2. Place apple halves on a baking sheet.
3. Sprinkle cinnamon over the apples and top with chopped walnuts.
4. Drizzle honey over the top.
5. Bake for 20-25 minutes until apples are tender.
6. Serve warm and savor the comforting flavors.

Nutrition Information:

- Calories: 180
- Protein: 2g
- Carbohydrates: 30g
- Fat: 8g
- Fiber: 6g
- Antioxidants: Moderate
- Portion Size: 1 serving

# Greek Yogurt and Honey Frozen Popsicles

Ingredients:

- 1 cup Greek yogurt
- 2 tablespoons honey
- 1/2 cup mixed berries (strawberries, blueberries, raspberries)

Instructions:

1. In a bowl, mix Greek yogurt and honey until well combined.
2. Spoon the mixture into popsicle molds, alternating with layers of mixed berries.
3. Insert popsicle sticks and freeze for at least 4 hours.
4. Unmold and enjoy these refreshing and creamy popsicles!

Nutrition Information:

- Calories: 120
- Protein: 8g
- Carbohydrates: 18g
- Fat: 2g

- Fiber: 2g
- Antioxidants: High
- Portion Size: 1 serving

## Turmeric and Ginger Infused Fruit Salad

Ingredients:

- 2 cups mixed fruits (pineapple, mango, kiwi, berries)
- 1 teaspoon turmeric powder
- 1 teaspoon fresh ginger, grated
- 1 tablespoon honey

Instructions:

1. In a bowl, combine mixed fruits.
2. Sprinkle turmeric powder and grated ginger over the fruits.
3. Drizzle honey and gently toss to coat.
4. Chill for 30 minutes before serving.
5. Delight in the vibrant colors and flavors.

Nutrition Information:

- Calories: 100
- Protein: 1g
- Carbohydrates: 25g
- Fat: 0.5g
- Fiber: 4g
- Antioxidants: High
- Portion Size: 1 serving

## Pumpkin Pie Energy Bites

Ingredients:

- 1 cup rolled oats
- 1/2 cup pumpkin puree
- 1/4 cup almond butter
- 1/4 cup honey
- 1 teaspoon pumpkin pie spice
- 1/4 cup chopped pecans

Instructions:

1. In a bowl, combine rolled oats, pumpkin puree, almond butter, honey, and pumpkin pie spice.
2. Fold in chopped pecans.

3. Roll the mixture into bite-sized balls.

4. Refrigerate for at least 1 hour before serving.

5. Enjoy these energy-packed pumpkin pie bites!

Nutrition Information:

- Calories: 120

- Protein: 3g

- Carbohydrates: 15g

- Fat: 6g

- Fiber: 2g

- Antioxidants: Moderate

- Portion Size: 2 bites

## Mixed Berry Sorbet

Ingredients:

- 2 cups mixed berries (strawberries, blueberries, raspberries)

- 1 tablespoon honey

- 1 tablespoon lemon juice

Instructions:

1.  Blend mixed berries, honey, and lemon juice until smooth.
2.  Pour the mixture into a shallow dish.
3.  Freeze for 3-4 hours, stirring every hour.
4.  Scoop and serve this refreshing mixed berry sorbet.

Nutrition Information:

- Calories: 80
- Protein: 1g
- Carbohydrates: 20g
- Fat: 0.5g
- Fiber: 5g
- Antioxidants: High
- Portion Size: 1 serving

## Almond Flour Banana Bread

Ingredients:

- 2 ripe bananas, mashed
- 2 cups almond flour
- 3 eggs
- 1/4 cup coconut oil, melted

- 1 teaspoon vanilla extract
- 1 teaspoon baking soda

Instructions:

1. Preheat the oven to 350°F (175°C).
2. In a bowl, mix mashed bananas, almond flour, eggs, melted coconut oil, vanilla extract, and baking soda.
3. Pour the batter into a greased loaf pan.
4. Bake for 40-45 minutes until golden brown.
5. Allow it to cool before slicing and savoring this almond flour banana bread.

Nutrition Information:

- Calories: 180
- Protein: 7g
- Carbohydrates: 15g
- Fat: 12g
- Fiber: 3g
- Antioxidants: Moderate
- Portion Size: 1 slice

# Avocado Chocolate Mousse

Ingredients:

- 2 ripe avocados
- 1/4 cup cocoa powder
- 1/4 cup maple syrup
- 1 teaspoon vanilla extract
- Pinch of sea salt

Instructions:

1. In a blender, combine avocados, cocoa powder, maple syrup, vanilla extract, and a pinch of sea salt.
2. Blend until smooth and creamy.
3. Refrigerate for at least 30 minutes before serving.
4. Indulge in the rich and velvety texture of this guilt-free avocado chocolate mousse.

Nutrition Information:

- Calories: 220
- Protein: 3g
- Carbohydrates: 20g
- Fat: 15g
- Fiber: 7g

- Antioxidants: Moderate
- Portion Size: 1 serving

## Pistachio and Cranberry Quinoa Bars

Ingredients:
- 1 cup cooked quinoa
- 1/2 cup pistachios, chopped
- 1/4 cup dried cranberries
- 1/4 cup honey
- 1/4 cup almond butter
- 1 teaspoon vanilla extract

Instructions:
1. In a bowl, mix cooked quinoa, chopped pistachios, dried cranberries, honey, almond butter, and vanilla extract.
2. Press the mixture into a lined baking dish.
3. Refrigerate for 2 hours before cutting into bars.
4. Enjoy these nutrient-packed pistachio and cranberry quinoa bars!

Nutrition Information:

- Calories: 180
- Protein: 5g
- Carbohydrates: 20g
- Fat: 9g
- Fiber: 3g
- Antioxidants: High
- Portion Size: 1 bar

## Lemon Poppy Seed Muffins

Ingredients:

- 2 cups almond flour
- 3 eggs
- 1/4 cup coconut oil, melted
- 1/4 cup honey
- Zest and juice of 2 lemons
- 1 tablespoon poppy seeds
- 1 teaspoon baking powder

Instructions:

1. Preheat the oven to 350°F (175°C).

2.  In a bowl, mix almond flour, eggs, melted coconut oil, honey, lemon zest, lemon juice, poppy seeds, and baking powder.

3.  Spoon the batter into muffin cups.

4.  Bake for 20-25 minutes until golden brown.

5.  Let them cool before enjoying these delightful lemon poppy seed muffins.

Nutrition Information:

- Calories: 150
- Protein: 6g
- Carbohydrates: 12g
- Fat: 10g
- Fiber: 3g
- Antioxidants: Moderate
- Portion Size: 1 muffin

## Cinnamon Roasted Sweet Potatoes

Ingredients:

- 2 sweet potatoes, peeled and cubed
- 1 tablespoon coconut oil, melted
- 1 teaspoon cinnamon

- 1 tablespoon maple syrup



Instructions:

1. Preheat the oven to 400°F (200°C).

2. In a bowl, toss sweet potato cubes with melted coconut oil and cinnamon.

3. Spread the sweet potatoes on a baking sheet.

4. Roast for 25-30 minutes until tender.

5. Drizzle maple syrup over the top before serving.

6. Enjoy the natural sweetness of cinnamon-roasted sweet potatoes.

Nutrition Information:

- Calories: 120

- Protein: 2g

- Carbohydrates: 25g

- Fat: 2g

- Fiber: 4g

- Antioxidants: Moderate

- Portion Size: 1 serving

# Blueberry Coconut Ice Cream

Ingredients:

- 2 cups frozen blueberries
- 1 can (14 oz) coconut milk
- 1/4 cup honey
- 1 teaspoon vanilla extract

Instructions:

1. Blend frozen blueberries, coconut milk, honey, and vanilla extract until smooth.
2. Pour the mixture into a container and freeze for 4-6 hours.
3. Scoop and enjoy this creamy and dairy-free blueberry coconut ice cream.

Nutrition Information:

- Calories: 150
- Protein: 1g
- Carbohydrates: 20g
- Fat: 8g
- Fiber: 3g
- Antioxidants: High

- Portion Size: 1 serving

## Pomegranate and Walnut Stuffed Dates

Ingredients:

- 15 Medjool dates, pitted
- 1/2 cup pomegranate seeds
- 1/4 cup walnuts, chopped
- 1 teaspoon cinnamon

Instructions:

1. In a bowl, mix pomegranate seeds, chopped walnuts, and cinnamon.
2. Stuff each date with the pomegranate and walnut mixture.
3. Arrange on a serving platter and enjoy these naturally sweet delights.

Nutrition Information:

- Calories: 120
- Protein: 2g

- Carbohydrates: 25g

- Fat: 4g

- Fiber: 3g

- Antioxidants: High

- Portion Size: 1 serving

# Chapter 7: Smoothies

Embarking on a journey towards a healthier lifestyle is a delightful exploration, and Chapter 7 brings you a symphony of flavors in the form of invigorating smoothie recipes. Packed with vibrant colors and bursting with nutrition, these concoctions not only tantalize the taste buds but also contribute to your anti-inflammatory goals.

## Green Goddess Detox Smoothie

Ingredients:

- 1 cup fresh spinach leaves
- 1/2 cucumber, peeled and sliced
- 1 green apple, cored and diced
- 1/2 lemon, juiced
- 1 cup coconut water
- Ice cubes (optional)

Instructions:

1. Combine spinach, cucumber, green apple, and lemon juice in a blender.

2. Add coconut water and blend until smooth.

3. If desired, add ice cubes and blend again for a refreshing chill.

Nutrition Information:

- Calories: 120
- Protein: 3g
- Carbohydrates: 25g
- Fat: 1g
- Fiber: 6g
- Antioxidants: High
- Portion Size: 1 serving

## Pineapple Turmeric Smoothie

Ingredients:

- 1 cup pineapple chunks
- 1 teaspoon turmeric powder
- 1/2 cup Greek yogurt
- 1 tablespoon chia seeds
- 1/2 cup almond milk
- Honey to taste

Instructions:

1. Blend pineapple, turmeric powder, Greek yogurt, and chia seeds until smooth.

2. Add almond milk gradually, adjusting thickness as desired.

3. Sweeten with honey to taste.

Nutrition Information:

- Calories: 150
- Protein: 5g
- Carbohydrates: 20g
- Fat: 6g
- Fiber: 8g
- Antioxidants: Moderate
- Portion Size: 1 serving

## Berry Blast Anti-Inflammatory Smoothie

Ingredients:

- 1/2 cup mixed berries (blueberries, strawberries, raspberries)

- 1/2 cup kale leaves, stems removed
- 1 tablespoon flaxseeds
- 1/2 cup pomegranate juice
- 1/2 cup water
- Ice cubes (optional)

Instructions:

1. Combine mixed berries, kale, and flaxseeds in a blender.
2. Pour in pomegranate juice and water, then blend until smooth.
3. Add ice cubes for an extra chill.

Nutrition Information:

- Calories: 90
- Protein: 4g
- Carbohydrates: 15g
- Fat: 2g
- Fiber: 5g
- Antioxidants: High
- Portion Size: 1 serving

# Mango and Ginger Smoothie

Ingredients:

- 1 cup ripe mango chunks
- 1 teaspoon freshly grated ginger
- 1/2 cup plain yogurt
- 1 tablespoon hemp seeds
- 1/2 cup coconut water
- Ice cubes (optional)

Instructions:

1. Blend mango chunks, grated ginger, yogurt, and hemp seeds until creamy.
2. Gradually add coconut water, adjusting thickness to preference.
3. Include ice cubes for an extra refreshing kick.

Nutrition Information:

- Calories: 140
- Protein: 6g
- Carbohydrates: 18g
- Fat: 5g
- Fiber: 4g

- Antioxidants: Moderate
- Portion Size: 1 serving

## Spinach and Blueberry Power Smoothie

Ingredients:

- 1 cup fresh blueberries
- 1 cup spinach leaves
- 1/2 banana
- 1 tablespoon almond butter
- 1/2 cup almond milk
- Ice cubes (optional)

Instructions:

1. Combine blueberries, spinach, banana, and almond butter in a blender.
2. Pour in almond milk and blend until smooth.
3. Add ice cubes for a cooler texture.

Nutrition Information:

- Calories: 160

- Protein: 5g

- Carbohydrates: 22g

- Fat: 7g

- Fiber: 6g

- Antioxidants: High

- Portion Size: 1 serving

## Golden Glow Tropical Smoothie

Ingredients:

- 1/2 cup pineapple chunks

- 1/2 cup mango chunks

- 1 teaspoon turmeric powder

- 1/2 cup coconut milk

- 1 tablespoon chia seeds

- Ice cubes (optional)

Instructions:

1. Blend pineapple, mango, turmeric powder, and coconut milk until smooth.

2. Add chia seeds and blend for an extra nutrient boost.

3. Include ice cubes for a refreshing twist.

Nutrition Information:

- Calories: 130
- Protein: 4g
- Carbohydrates: 18g
- Fat: 6g
- Fiber: 5g
- Antioxidants: High
- Portion Size: 1 serving

## Kale and Pineapple Smoothie

Ingredients:

- 1 cup kale leaves, stems removed
- 1/2 cup pineapple chunks
- 1/2 cucumber, peeled and sliced
- 1 tablespoon flaxseeds
- 1/2 cup coconut water
- Ice cubes (optional)

Instructions:

1. Blend kale, pineapple, cucumber, and flaxseeds until well combined.
2. Gradually add coconut water and blend until smooth.

3.  Introduce ice cubes for a cooler sensation.

Nutrition Information:

- Calories: 110
- Protein: 4g
- Carbohydrates: 16g
- Fat: 4g
- Fiber: 5g
- Antioxidants: Moderate
- Portion Size: 1 serving

## Coconut Water and Berry Smoothie

Ingredients:

- 1/2 cup mixed berries (strawberries, raspberries, blackberries)
- 1/2 cup coconut water
- 1/2 cup Greek yogurt
- 1 tablespoon chia seeds
- 1/2 banana
- Ice cubes (optional)

Instructions:

1.  Blend mixed berries, coconut water, Greek yogurt, and chia seeds until smooth.

2.  Add banana and blend again until creamy.

3.  Consider adding ice cubes for a chilled delight.

Nutrition Information:

- Calories: 120
- Protein: 5g
- Carbohydrates: 18g
- Fat: 3g
- Fiber: 6g
- Antioxidants: High
- Portion Size: 1 serving

## Cucumber Mint Cooler Smoothie

Ingredients:

- 1/2 cucumber, peeled and sliced
- 1/2 cup fresh mint leaves
- 1/2 lemon, juiced
- 1 tablespoon honey
- 1/2 cup coconut water

- Ice cubes (optional)

Instructions:

1. Blend cucumber, mint leaves, lemon juice, and honey until well combined.
2. Pour in coconut water gradually and blend for a smooth texture.
3. Add ice cubes for an extra refreshing experience.

Nutrition Information:

- Calories: 80
- Protein: 1g
- Carbohydrates: 20g
- Fat: 0g
- Fiber: 3g
- Antioxidants: Moderate
- Portion Size: 1 serving

# Avocado and Spinach Protein Smoothie

Ingredients:

- 1/2 avocado, peeled and pitted
- 1 cup fresh spinach leaves
- 1/2 cup plain Greek yogurt
- 1 scoop protein powder (vanilla or unflavored)
- 1/2 cup almond milk
- Ice cubes (optional)

Instructions:

1. Blend avocado, spinach, Greek yogurt, and protein powder until creamy.
2. Gradually add almond milk, adjusting thickness to preference.
3. Include ice cubes for a cool and satisfying texture.

Nutrition Information:

- Calories: 180
- Protein: 15g
- Carbohydrates: 10g
- Fat: 10g

- Fiber: 5g

- Antioxidants: Moderate

- Portion Size: 1 serving

# Almond Butter Banana Bliss Smoothie

Ingredients:

- 1/2 banana

- 1 tablespoon almond butter

- 1/2 cup almond milk

- 1 tablespoon flaxseeds

- 1/2 teaspoon cinnamon

- Ice cubes (optional)

Instructions:

1. Blend banana, almond butter, almond milk, flaxseeds, and cinnamon until smooth.

2. Adjust thickness by adding more almond milk if needed.

3. Include ice cubes for a refreshing and nutty flavor.

Nutrition Information:

- Calories: 200
- Protein: 7g
- Carbohydrates: 20g
- Fat: 12g
- Fiber: 6g
- Antioxidants: Moderate
- Portion Size: 1 serving

## Cherry Almond Anti-Inflammatory Smoothie

Ingredients:

- 1/2 cup frozen cherries
- 1/4 cup almonds
- 1/2 cup Greek yogurt
- 1 tablespoon chia seeds
- 1/2 cup coconut water
- Ice cubes (optional)

Instructions:

1.  Blend frozen cherries, almonds, Greek yogurt, and chia seeds until well combined.
2.  Pour in coconut water gradually, adjusting thickness as desired.
3.  Add ice cubes for a chilled and satisfying treat.

Nutrition Information:

- Calories: 150
- Protein: 6g
- Carbohydrates: 18g
- Fat: 7g
- Fiber: 4g
- Antioxidants: High
- Portion Size: 1 serving

## Turmeric and Orange Citrus Smoothie

Ingredients:

- 1/2 teaspoon turmeric powder
- 1 orange, peeled and segmented

- 1/2 cup pineapple chunks
- 1/2 cup Greek yogurt
- 1/2 cup water
- Ice cubes (optional)

Instructions:

1. Blend turmeric powder, orange segments, pineapple chunks, and Greek yogurt until smooth.
2. Gradually add water, adjusting thickness to your liking.
3. Include ice cubes for an extra refreshing twist.

Nutrition Information:

- Calories: 130
- Protein: 5g
- Carbohydrates: 20g
- Fat: 3g
- Fiber: 4g
- Antioxidants: High
- Portion Size: 1 serving

# Beetroot and Berry Elixir Smoothie

Ingredients:

- 1/2 cup cooked and peeled beetroot
- 1/2 cup mixed berries (strawberries, raspberries, blackberries)
- 1/2 cup coconut water
- 1 tablespoon hemp seeds
- 1/2 banana
- Ice cubes (optional)

Instructions:

1. Blend cooked beetroot, mixed berries, coconut water, and hemp seeds until well combined.
2. Add banana and blend again for a creamy texture.
3. Consider including ice cubes for a cool and vibrant elixir.

Nutrition Information:

- Calories: 140
- Protein: 5g
- Carbohydrates: 18g
- Fat: 6g

- Fiber: 5g

- Antioxidants: High

- Portion Size: 1 serving

## Chocolate Protein Powerhouse Smoothie

Ingredients:

- 1 scoop chocolate protein powder

- 1 tablespoon almond butter

- 1/2 cup almond milk

- 1/2 banana

- 1 tablespoon cacao powder

- Ice cubes (optional)

Instructions:

1. Blend chocolate protein powder, almond butter, almond milk, banana, and cacao powder until smooth.

2. Adjust thickness by adding more almond milk if needed.

3. Add ice cubes for a rich and indulgent texture.

Nutrition Information:

- Calories: 220
- Protein: 20g
- Carbohydrates: 15g
- Fat: 10g
- Fiber: 6g
- Antioxidants: Low
- Portion Size: 1 serving

# CONCLUSION

As you reflect on the knowledge gained from the insightful introduction, the structured 28-day meal plan, and the diverse recipes spanning breakfast to desserts and smoothies, remember that this isn't just a diet; it's a holistic lifestyle shift. The incorporation of anti-inflammatory ingredients isn't merely about what you eat; it's about nourishing your body, mind, and spirit.

By embracing this approach, you're not just adopting a healthier way of eating; you're fostering a sustainable relationship with your body. Each recipe is a testament to the idea that healthful eating can be a gratifying experience, a symphony of flavors and textures that contributes to your overall vitality.

The 28-day journey outlined in this book is not a strict regimen but rather a flexible guide tailored to your unique preferences and dietary needs. It encourages you to explore, experiment, and savor the joy of preparing and consuming nourishing meals. It's about understanding your body's responses, recognizing the impact of food on your energy levels, and appreciating the intricate dance between nutrition and well-being.

As you take the knowledge and recipes provided within these pages into your daily life, we hope you discover not just a diet but a sustainable lifestyle that promotes longevity and vitality. Embrace the culinary adventure, relish the flavors, and witness the positive changes in your body as it reaps the benefits of anti-inflammatory nutrition.

Remember, this is a journey, and every step counts. Your commitment to nourishing yourself with these wholesome, anti-inflammatory recipes is a powerful stride toward a healthier and more vibrant you. May this book be a constant companion, inspiring you to make mindful choices that resonate with your body's needs, ultimately leading you to a state of balanced well-being.

Here's to your health, happiness, and the beginning of a lifelong love affair with nutritious and delicious living!

www.ingramcontent.com/pod-product-compliance
Lightning Source LLC
Chambersburg PA
CBHW071604270726
48661CB00018B/1174